NATURALLY

KETO

Traditional Food Favorites
for a Low-Carb Lifestyle

RYAN BERG

© Copyright 2021 - All rights reserved.

TABLE OF CONTENTS

REFRESHING DRINKS AND SMOOTHIES 98

KETO KITCHEN STAPLES AND DISH RECIPES 111

BREAKFAST

1 - Spanish Omelet

Preparation	Cooking	Servings
12 min	12 min	6

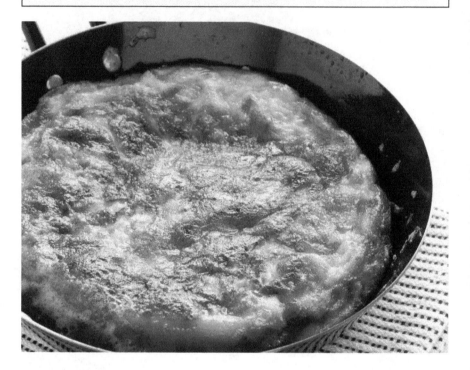

Ingredients

- 4 eggs
- Cayenne or black pepper
- 1 Cup finely chopped vegetables of your choosing.

Direction

1. In a pan on high heat, stir-fry the vegetables in extra virgin olive oil until lightly crispy.

2. Cook the eggs with one tablespoon of water and a pinch of pepper.
3. When almost cooked, top with the vegetables and flip to cook briefly.
4. Serve

Per Serving: Calories: 145Fat: 13g Carbohydrates: 4.6g Protein: 7.5g

2 - Breakfast Sausage Casserole

Preparation	Cooking	Servings
12 min	40 min	6

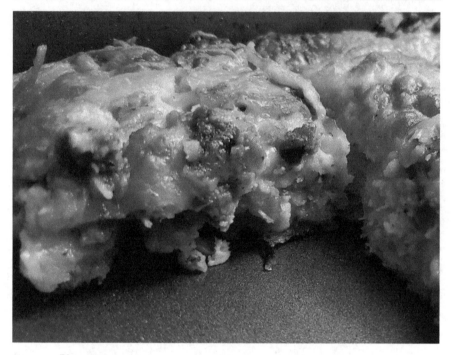

Ingredients

- 6 eggs, beaten
- 1 head chopped cauliflower
- 2 lb sausage, cooked and crumbled
- 3 cups heavy whipping cream
- 2 cup sharp cheddar cheese, grated

Direction

1. Cook the sausage as usual.

2. In a large bowl, mix the sausage, heavy whipping cream, chopped cauliflower, cheese, and eggs.
3. Pour into a greased casserole dish.
4. Cook for 45 minutes at 350°F/175°C, or until firm.
5. Top with cheese and serve.

Per Serving: Calories: 260 Fat: 24.2g Carbohydrates: 1.5g Protein: 11.9g

3 - Scrambled Mug Eggs

Preparation	Cooking	Servings
12 min	**6 min**	**6**

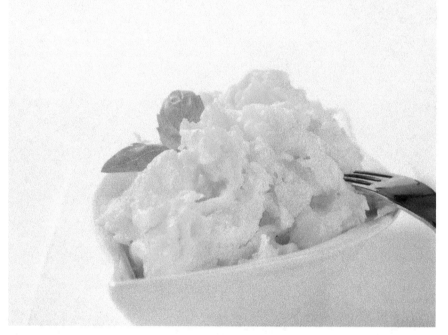

Ingredients

- 2 mug
- 4 eggs
- Salt and pepper
- Shredded cheese
- Your favorite buffalo wing sauce

Direction

1. Crack the eggs into a mug and whisk until blended.

2. Put the mug into your microwave and cook for 1.5 - 2 minutes, depending on the power of your microwave.
3. Leave for a few minutes and remove from the microwave.
4. Sprinkle with salt and pepper. Add your desired amount of cheese on top.
5. Using a fork, mix everything together.
6. Then add your favorite buffalo or hot sauce and mix again.
7. Serve!

Per Serving: Calories: 334Fat: 32gCarbohydrates: 1.3g Protein: 11.6g

4 - Salmon Omelet

Preparation	Cooking	Servings
15 min	**8 min**	**6**

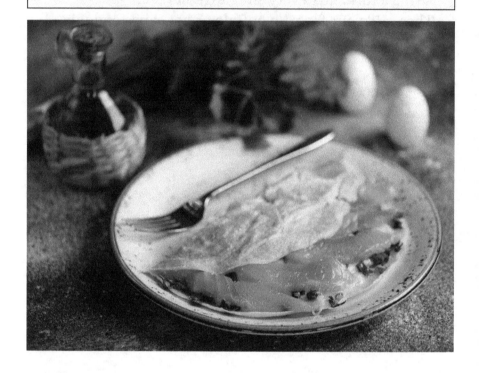

Ingredients

- 6 eggs
- 2 smoked salmon
- 6 links beef sausage
- 1/2 cup onions
- 1/2 cup provolone cheese

Direction

1. Whisk the eggs and pour them into a skillet.
2. Follow the standard method for making an omelet.
3. Add the onions, salmon, and cheese before turning the omelet over.
4. Sprinkle the omelet with cheese and serve with the sausages on the side.
5. Serve!

Per Serving: Calories: 480 Carbohydrates: 2.2g Protein: 38g

5 – Eggs with Spinach and Cheese

Preparation	Cooking	Servings
10 min	25 min	6

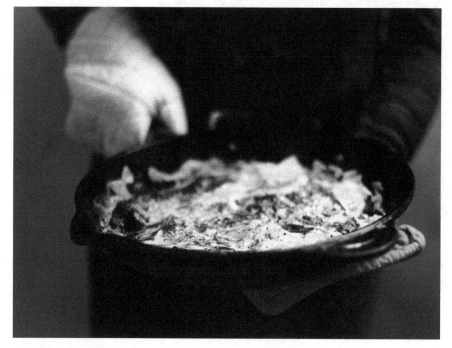

Ingredients

- 6 whole eggs
- 4 oz cottage cheese
- 3-4 oz chopped spinach 1/4 cup parmesan cheese 1/2 cup of milk

Direction

1. Preheat your oven to 375°F/190°C.

2. In a large bowl, whisk the eggs, cottage cheese, parmesan, and milk.
3. Mix in the spinach.
4. Transfer to a small, greased oven dish.
5. Sprinkle the cheese on top.
6. Bake for 25-30 minutes.
7. Let cool for 5 minutes and serve.
8. Serve!

Per Serving: Calories: 190 Fat: 24g Carbohydrates: 2.3g Protein: 15.3g

APPETIZERS

6 - Shortbread

Preparation	Cooking	Servings
15 min	**18 min**	**4**

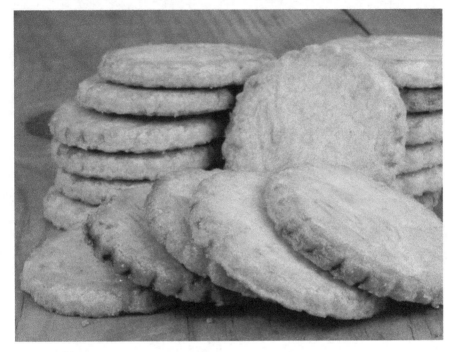

Ingredients

- ½ cup Erythritol
- 1 teaspoon vanilla extract
- 2 and ½ cups almond flour
- 6 tablespoons butter

Direction

1. Pre-heat your oven to 350 degrees F.

2. Line cookie sheet with parchment paper.

3. Take a bowl and beat in butter, Erythritol and mix until it is fluffy.

4. Beat in vanilla extract, beat in almond flour ½ cup at a time.

5. Use a tablespoon to transfer the dough to a cookie sheet.

6. Flatten each cookie to about 1/3 inch thick.

7. Bake for 12-15 minutes until golden.

8. Let them cool and serve

9. Enjoy!

Per Serving: Calories: 134 Fat: 11g Carbohydrates: 1g Protein: 2g

7 - Keto Muffin

Preparation	Cooking	Servings
15 min	**2 min**	**6**

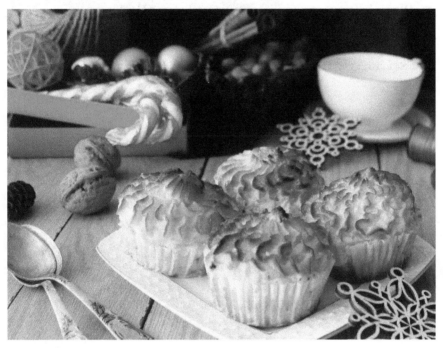

Ingredients

- 2 whole egg
- 3 teaspoon coconut flour
- A pinch of baking soda
- A pinch salt
- Coconut oil, for grease

Direction

1. Grease ramekin dish with coconut oil.
2. Keep it aside.
3. Take a bowl and add ingredients and mix well.
4. Pour batter into a ramekin.
5. Place into microwave for 1 minute on HIGH.
6. Serve and enjoy!

Per Serving: Calories: 112 Fat: 5.2g Carbohydrates: 3.1g Protein: 7.3g

8 - Lemon Cheesecake no Bake

Preparation	Cooking	Servings
70 min	0 min	8

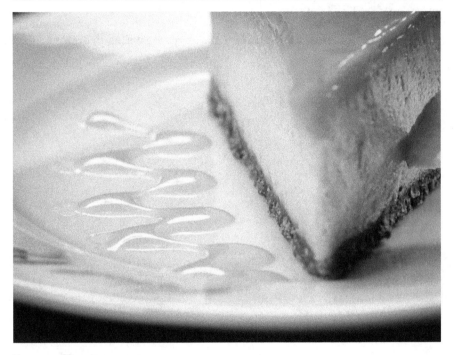

Ingredients

- 10 ounces cream cheese

- 4 ounces full-fat cream

- 2 tablespoon lemon juice

- Few drops of vanilla extract

- Peel 1 lemon, grated

Direction

1. Add cream, cream cheese, and mix well.

2. Add the remaining ingredients.

3. Transfer the mixture to your fridge.

4. Keep it for 1 hour in the fridge.

5. Serve and enjoy!

Per Serving: Calories: 210 Fat: 16g Carbohydrates: 2.2g Protein: 6.1g

9 - Vegetable Quiche

Preparation	Cooking	Servings
15 min	**30 min**	**8**

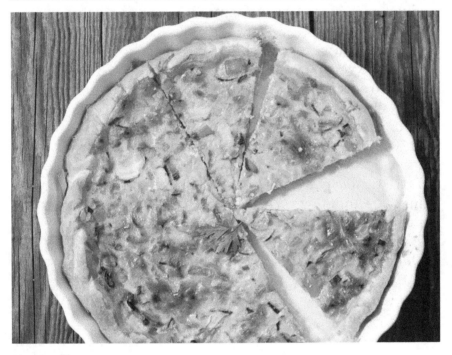

<u>Ingredients</u>

- 2 tablespoon melted butter, divided
- 8 eggs
- 4 ounces (85 g) goat cheese, divided
- 4 cup heavy whipping cream
- 2 scallion, white and green parts, chopped
- 1 cup mushrooms, sliced
- 12cup fresh spinach, chopped
- 16 cherry tomatoes, cut in half

Direction

1. Preheat the oven to 350°F (180²C). Coat a pie pan with ¹/2 teaspoon of melted butter and set aside.

2. Whisk together the eggs, 2 ounces (57 g) of goat cheese, and heavy whipping cream in a bowl until creamy and smooth, you can use a blender to make it easier. Set aside.

3. Heat the remaining butter in a nonstick skillet over medium-high heat. Add and saute scallion and mushrooms for 2 minutes or until tender. Add and saute the spinach for another 2 minutes or until softened.

4. Pour the vegetable mixture into the pie pan, and use a spatula to spread the mixture so it covers the bottom of the pan evenly.

5. Pour the egg mixture over the vegetable mixture. Top them with the cherry tomato halves and remaining goat cheese.

6. Place the pie pan in the preheated oven and bake for 20 minutes or until fluffy. You can check the doneness by cutting a small slit in the center, if raw eggs run into the cut, then baking for another few minutes.

7. Divide the quiche among four platters and serve warm.

Per Serving: Calories: 385 Fat: 33g Carbohydrates: 4.2g Protein: 19g

10 - Rutabaga Cakes

Preparation	Cooking	Servings
15 min	30 min	8

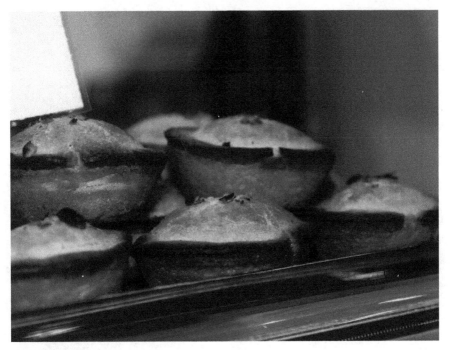

Ingredients

- 4 rutabagas, thinly sliced
- 1 stick butter, melted
- 4 tablespoons fresh thyme, chopped
- 4 teaspoons salt

Direction

1. Place a saucepan over medium heat.

2. Add butter and let it melt.

3. Add thyme and stir for 2 minutes.

4. Take a bowl and add rutabaga slices into it and pour the mix.

5. Layer rutabaga slices in muffin tins and top with butter on top.

6. Take a foil and cover muffin tins.

7. Preheat your oven to 350 degrees F.

8. Bake for 25-30 minutes.

9. Serve and enjoy!

Per Serving: Calories: 44 Fat: 3.3g Carbohydrates: 1.2g Protein: 0.6g

11 - Eggplant Fries		
Preparation	Cooking	Servings
15 min	20 min	6

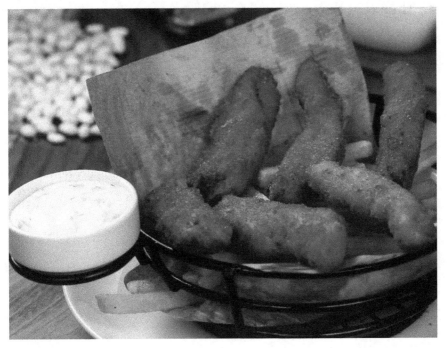

Ingredients

- 4 whole eggs
- 3 cups almond flour
- 3 tablespoons coconut oil, spray
- 3 eggplant, peeled and cut thinly
- Salt and pepper to taste

__Direction__

1. Preheat your oven to 400 degrees Fahrenheit.

2. Take a bowl and mix with salt and black pepper in it.

3. Take another bowl and beat eggs until frothy.

4. Dip the eggplant pieces into eggs.

5. Then coat them with a flour mixture.

6. Add another layer of flour and egg.

7. Then, take a baking sheet and grease with coconut oil on top.

8. Bake for about 15 minutes.

9. Serve and enjoy!

Per Serving: Calories: 245 Fat: 14.2g Carbohydrates: 3.9g Protein: 6.2g

12 - Avocado Stuffed Parmesan		
Preparation	Cooking	Servings
15 min	20 min	6

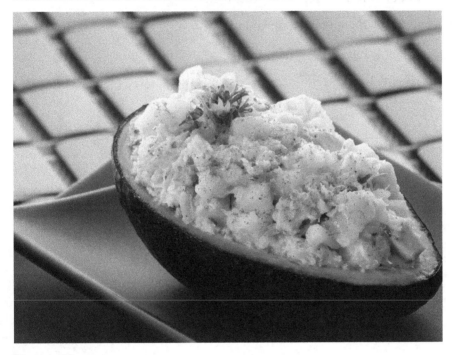

Ingredients

- 1 whole avocado
- 1 tablespoon chipotle sauce
- 1 tablespoon lime juice
- ¼ cup parmesan cheese
- Salt and pepper to taste

Direction

1. Prepare avocado by slicing half lengthwise and discard the seed.

2. Gently prick the skin of the avocado with a fork.

3. Set your avocado halves, skin down on the small baking sheet lined with aluminum foil.

4. Top with sauce and drizzle lime juice.

5. Season with salt and pepper.

6. Sprinkle half parmesan cheese in each cavity, set your broiler to high for 2 minutes.

7. Add rest of the cheese and return to your broiler until cheese melts and avocado slightly browns.

8. Serve hot and enjoy!

Per Serving: Calories: 31 Fat: 40.2g Carbohydrates: 7.3g Protein: 5.2g

BEEF

13 - Filet Mignon Dijon Sauce

Preparation	Cooking	Servings
15 min	**15 min**	4

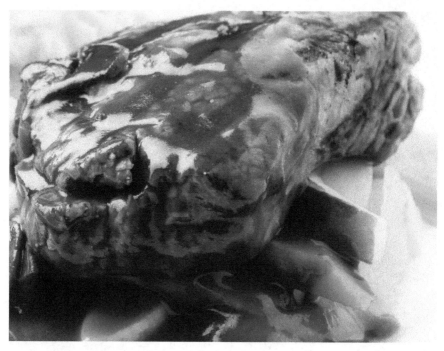

Ingredients

- 2 teaspoons lard, at room temperature
- 2 pounds beef filet mignon, cut into bite-sized chunks
- Flaky salt and ground black pepper, to season
- 1 tablespoon Dijon mustard
- 1 cup double cream

Direction

1. Melt the lard in a saucepan over moderate heat; now, sear the filet mignon for 2 to 3 minutes per side— season with salt and pepper to taste.
2. Fold in the Dijon mustard and cream. Reduce the heat to medium-low and continue to cook for a further 6 minutes or until the sauce has reduced slightly.
3. Serve in individual plates, garnished with cauli rice if desired. Enjoy!

Per Serving: Calories: 311 Fat: 2.2g Carbohydrates: 2.1g Protein: 37g

14 - Beef Dish Shitake Butter

Preparation	Cooking	Servings
15 min	10 min	6

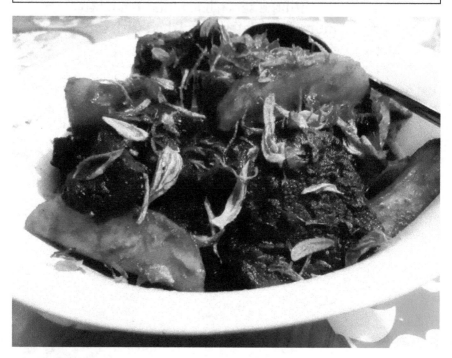

Ingredients

- 2 cups shitake mushrooms, sliced
- 4 ribeye steaks
- 2 tbsp butter
- 2 tsp olive oil
- Salt and black pepper to taste

Direction

1. Heat olive oil in a pan over medium heat. Rub the steaks with salt and pepper and cook for 4 minutes per side. Set aside.
2. Melt butter in the pan and cook the shitakes for 4 minutes.
3. Pour the butter and mushrooms over the steak.

Per Serving: Calories: 317 Fat: 30g Carbohydrates: 3.2g Protein: 31g

15 - Beef Meatballs

Preparation	Cooking	Servings
15 min	20 min	6

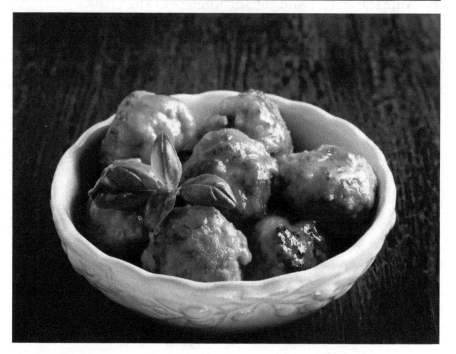

Ingredients

- 2 lb ground beef
- 1 cup grated parmesan cheese
- 2 tbsp minced garlic (or paste)
- 1 cup mozzarella cheese
- 1 tsp freshly ground pepper

Direction

1. Preheat your oven to 400°F/200°C.

2. In a bowl, mix all the ingredients together.
3. Roll the meat mixture into 6 generous meatballs.
4. Bake inside your oven at 170°F/80°C for about 18 minutes.
5. Serve with sauce!

Per Serving: Calories: 377 Fat: 21g Carbohydrates: 1.8g Protein: 16g

PORK

16 - Oven Baked Pork Shoulder

Preparation	Cooking	Servings
15 min	**10 hours**	**8**

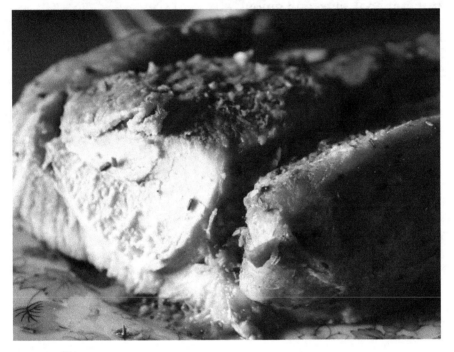

Ingredients

- 8 pounds pork shoulder
- 4 teaspoons oregano
- 2 teaspoon garlic powder
- 2 teaspoon onion powder
- Salt and pepper to taste

Direction

1. Pre-heat your oven to 250-degree F

2. Rinse meat and wash well, rub the meat with seasoning

3. Take a roasting pan and cover with aluminum foil

4. Transfer meat to the pan

5. Cover with another foil and transfer to oven

6. Bake for 9-10 hours

7. Remove meat, increase oven temperature to 500-degree F

8. Return meat and bake for 15-20 minutes more

9. Let it cool, slice and enjoy!

Per Serving: Calories: 440 Fat: 34g Carbohydrates: 1.2g Protein: 32g

17 - Pork Chops Onion and Bacon

Preparation	Cooking	Servings
15 min	50 min	6

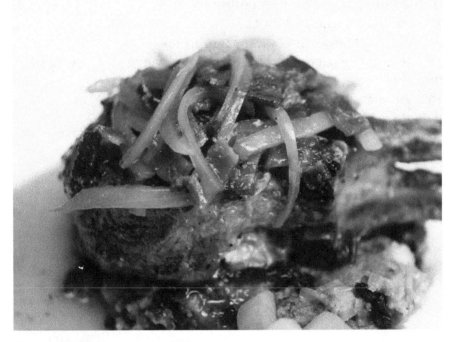

Ingredients

- 3 onions, peeled and chopped
- 6 bacon slices, chopped
- 1 cup chicken stock
- Salt and pepper to taste
- 6 pork chops

Direction

1. Heat up pan over medium-heat and add bacon

2. Stir and cook until crispy

3. Transfer to bowl

4. Return pan to medium heat and add onions, season with salt and pepper

5. Stir and cook for 15 minutes

6. Transfer to same bowl with bacon

7. Return the pan to heat (medium-high) and add pork chops

8. Season with salt and pepper and brown for 3 minutes

9. Flip and lower heat to medium

10. Cook for 7 minutes more

11. Add stock and stir cook for 2 minutes

12. Return the bacon and onions to the pan and stir cook for 1 minute

13. Serve and enjoy!

Per Serving: Calories: 315 Fat: 17g Carbohydrates: 6.2g Protein: 35g

POULTRY

18 - Duck Eye Ribeye

Preparation	Cooking	Servings
15 min	**20 min**	**6**

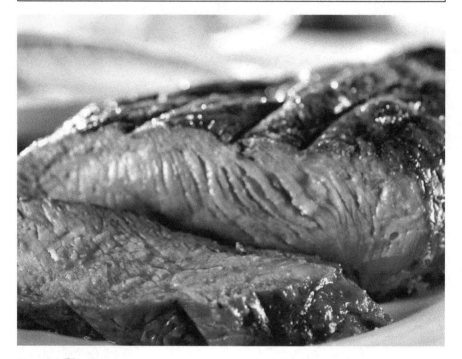

Ingredients

- One 16-oz ribeye steak (1 - 1 ¹14 inches thick)
- 2 tbsp duck fat (or other high smoke point oil like peanut oil)
- 1 tbsp butter
- 1 tsp thyme, chopped
- Salt and pepper to taste

Direction

1. Preheat a skillet in your oven at 400°F/200°C.
2. Season the steaks with oil, salt, and pepper. Remove the skillet from the oven once pre-heated.
3. Put the skillet on your stove top burner on medium heat and drizzle in the oil.
4. Sear the steak for 1-4 minutes, depending on if you like it rare, medium, or well done.
5. Turn over the steak and place it in your oven for 6 minutes.
6. Take out the steak from your oven and place it back on the stove top on low heat.
7. Toss in the butter and thyme and cook for 3 minutes, basting as you go along.
8. Rest for 5 minutes and serve.

Per Serving Calories: 720 Fat: 61g Carbohydrates: 2g Protein: 35g

19 - Turkey Avocado Rolls

Preparation	Cooking	Servings
15 min	**7 min**	**6**

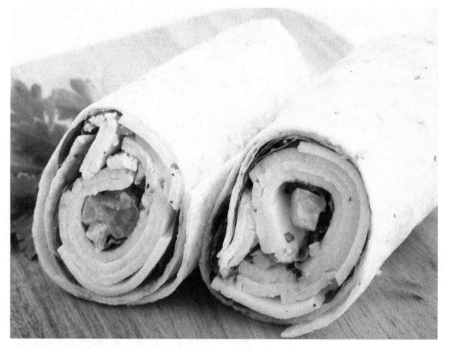

Ingredients

- 12 slices (12 oz) turkey breast
- 12 slices Swiss cheese
- 2 cups baby spinach
- 1 large avocado, cut into
- 12 slices
- 1 cup homemade mayonnaise

Direction

1. Lay out the slices of turkey breast flat and place a slice of Swiss cheese on top of each one.
2. Top each slice with 1 cup baby spinach and 3 slices of avocado.
3. Drizzle the mayonnaise on top.
4. Sprinkle each "sandwich" with lemon pepper.
5. Roll up the sandwiches and secure them with toothpicks.
6. Serve immediately or refrigerate until ready to serve.

Per Serving Calories: 140 Fat: 9.2g Carbohydrates: 5.3g Protein: 15.2g

20 - Savory Grilled Chicken

Preparation	Cooking	Servings
15 min	15 min	6

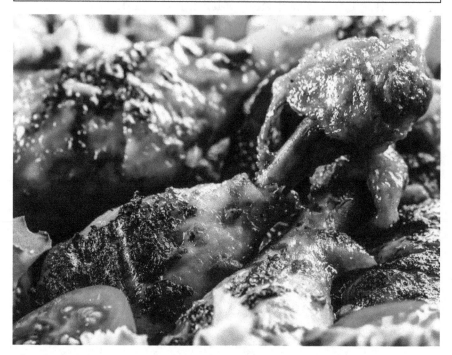

Ingredients

- 2 teaspoon dry mustard
- 2 teaspoon light brown sugar
- 2 teaspoon onion powder
- 4 pound skinless chicken breast
- Kosher salt & White pepper

Direction

1. Set the grill to preheat at medium-high temperatures as you add some greasing
2. In a small bowl, add onion powder, dry mustard, salt, brown sugar, and white pepper and mix well
3. Pass the chicken meat through the mixture to coat evenly.
4. Grill the chicken for 6 minutes on each side
5. Serve!

Per Serving Calories: 186 Fat: 4.3g Carbohydrates: 2.1g Protein: 34g

21 - Mediterranean Turkey Cutlets

Preparation	Cooking	Servings
15 min	15 min	6

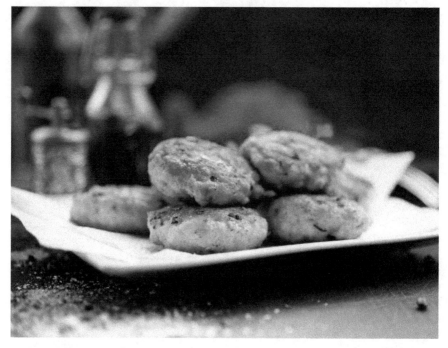

Ingredients

- 2 tablespoon olive oil
- 2 pound turkey cutlets
- 1/2 cup low carb flour mix
- 1 teaspoon Greek seasoning
- 1 teaspoon turmeric powder

Direction

1. In a medium bowl, mix the turkey cutlets with turmeric powder, low carb flour mix, and Greek seasoning
2. Put a frying pan on fire, then add the oil to heat.
3. Add the cutlets and cook for 5 minutes on each side under medium-low heat.
4. Serve!

Per Serving Calories: 293 Fat: 14g Carbohydrates: 4g Protein: 35g

FISH

22 - Cod and Tomato Capers

Preparation	Cooking	Servings
15 min	20 min	6

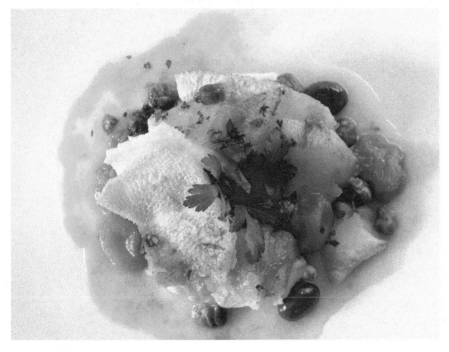

Ingredients

- 6 cod fillets, boneless
- 3 tablespoons avocado oil
- 2 cup tomato passata
- 3 tablespoons capers, drained
- 3 tablespoons parsley, chopped

Direction

1. In a roasting pan, combine the cod with the oil and the other ingredients, toss gently, introduce in the oven at 370 degrees F and bake for 25 minutes.
2. Divide between plates and serve

Per Serving Calories: 140 Fat: 3.2g Carbohydrates: 0.9g Protein: 4g

23 - Tuna Salad and Pickle Boats

Preparation	Cooking	Servings
40 min	**0 min**	**6**

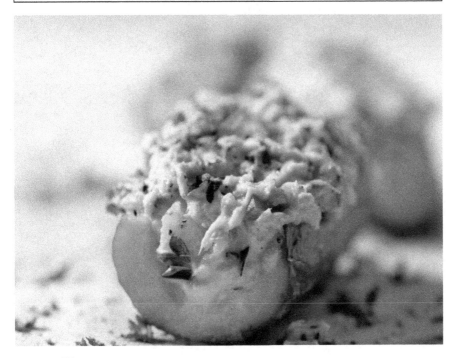

<u>Ingredients</u>

- 22 oz canned and drained tuna
- 6 large dill pickles
- 1/2 tsp garlic powder
- 1/3 cup sugar-free mayonnaise
- 1 tsp onion powder

Direction

1. Mix the mayo, tuna, onion, and garlic powders in a bowl. Cut the pickles in half, lengthwise. Top each half with a tuna mixture.

2. Place in the fridge for 30 minutes and serve

Per Serving Calories: 128 Fat: 12g Carbohydrates: 1.6g Protein: 10g

24 - Tuna and Spinach Salad

Preparation	Cooking	Servings
15 min	0 min	6

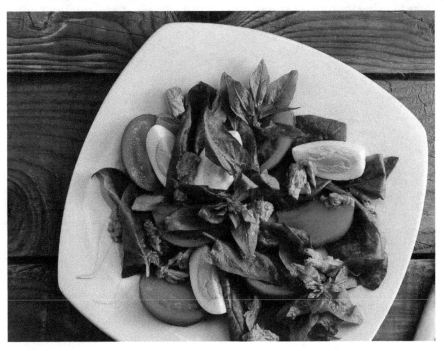

<u>Ingredients</u>

- 3 oz of spinach leaves
- 3 oz tuna, packed in water
- 1/2 tsp ground black pepper
- 1/2 tsp sea salt
- 3 tbsp coconut oil, melted

Direction

1. Take a salad bowl, place spinach leaves in it, drizzle with 1 tbsp oil, sprinkle with 1/8 tsp of salt and black pepper, and then toss until mixed.

2. Top with tuna, sprinkle with remaining salt and black pepper, drizzle with oil and then serve

Per Serving Calories: 145 Fat: 52g Carbohydrates: 1.2g Protein: 0.6g

SOUPS

25 - Spicy Fish Stew

Preparation	Cooking	Servings
20 min	30 min	8

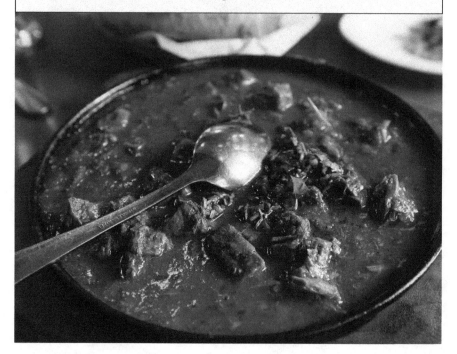

Ingredients

- 8 white fish fillets
- 2 cup vegetable stock
- 2 red and 1 green bell pepper, sliced
- 2 cup Marinara Tomato Sauce, low carb
- 2 green onion, sliced

Direction

1. Add vegetable stock, red bell pepper, green onion, sliced bell pepper, and green onion into your crockpot.

2. Mix them well.

3. Pour the tomato sauce.

4. Season it with salt and pepper.

5. Place the fish fillets and fill them with hot sauce carefully.

6. Cook for 6 hours on low heat.

7. Serve hot and enjoy!

Per Serving Calories: 240 Fat: 10g Carbohydrates: 7.2g Protein: 31g

26 - Minty Avocado Soup

Preparation	Cooking	Servings
20 min	**0 min**	**6**

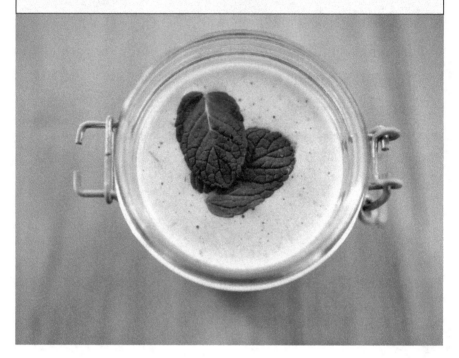

Ingredients

- 1 avocado, ripe
- 1 cup coconut milk, chilled
- 2 romaine lettuce leaves
- 20 mint leaves, fresh
- 1 tablespoon lime juice

Direction

1. Turn on your slow cooker and add all the ingredients into it.

2. Mix them in a food processor.

3. Make a smooth mixture.

4. Let it chill for 10 minutes.

5. Serve and enjoy!

Per Serving Calories: 270 Fat: 25 g Carbohydrates: 11g Protein: 4.2g

27 - Guacamole Soup

Preparation	Cooking	Servings
15 min	0 min	6

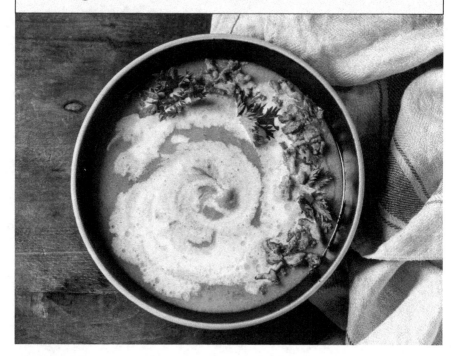

Ingredients

- 6 cups vegetable broth
- 3 ripe avocados, pitted
- 1 cup cilantro, freshly chopped
- 2 tomato, chopped
- 1 cup heavy cream

Direction

1   Add all the ingredients into a blender.

2   Blend until creamy by using an immersion blender.

3   Let it chill for 1 hour.

4   Serve and enjoy!

Per Serving Calories: 148 Fat: 15g Carbohydrates: 6.2g Protein: 7.2g

28 - Zucchini Soup

Preparation	Cooking	Servings
15 min	8 hours	8

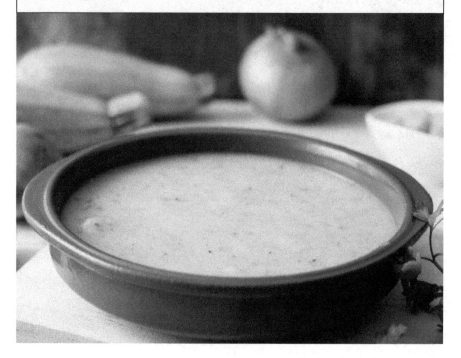

Ingredients

- 4 cups vegetable broth
- 4 zucchinis, cut in chunks
- 4 tablespoons sour cream, low fat
- 4 cloves garlic, minced
- Salt, pepper, thyme, and pepper, to taste

Direction

1. Add all the ingredients except sour cream to a crockpot.

2. Close the lid.

3. Cook for 6-8 hours on low.

4. Add sour cream.

5. Make a smooth puree by using a blender.

6. Serve hot with parmesan cheese if you want.

7. Enjoy!

Per Serving Calories: 70 Fat: 1.2g Carbohydrates: 8g Protein: 2.5g

DESSERTS

29 - Macadamia Fat Bomb

Preparation	Cooking	Servings
70 min	0 min	8

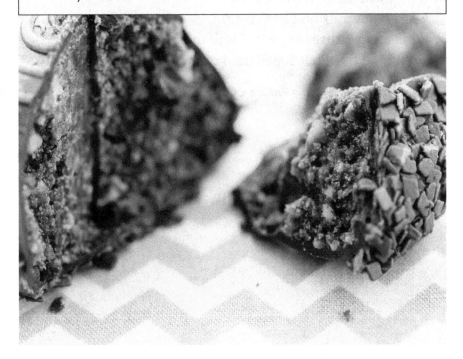

Ingredients

- 4 oz of unsweetened cocoa butter

- 4 tbsp of unsweetened cocoa powder

- 4 tbsp of Swerve

- 8 oz of macadamia, chopped

- 1/2 c of heavy cream

Direction

1. Melt in cocoa butter in a small saucepan over medium heat
2. Add cocoa powder to the saucepan
3. Add swerve, mix well until ingredients are blended well and melted
4. Add macadamias and stir
5. Add cream, mix and heat it up
6. Pour the mixture into Fat Bomb molds
7. Let it chill until hardened, and enjoy!

Per Serving Calories: 267 Fat: 28g Carbohydrates: 4g Protein: 3g

30 - Double Berry Ice Pops

Preparation	Cooking	Servings
2 hours	**0 min**	**8**

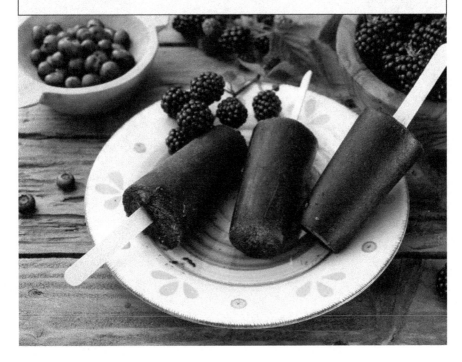

Ingredients

- 2 can use coconut cream

- 2 c of unsweetened full-fat coconut milk

- 8 drops liquid stevia

- 2 tsp of vanilla extract

- 2 c of mixed blueberries and blackberries

<u>Direction</u>

1. Take a food processor and add coconut cream, vanilla, and sweetener
2. Process well and add mixed berries, pulse for a few times
3. Pour into pop molds and freeze for 2 hours
4. Serve and enjoy!

Per Serving Calories: 145 Fat: 15g Carbohydrates: 2.2g Protein: 1.6g

31 - Dark Walnut Fudge

Preparation	Cooking	Servings
20 min	**0 min**	**8**

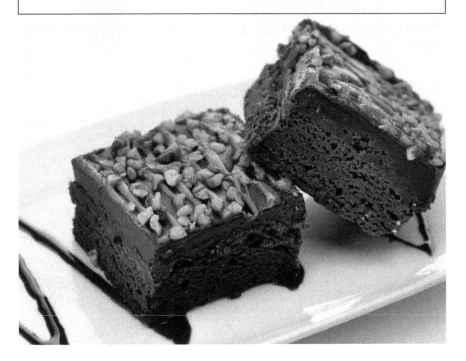

Ingredients

- 8 and ½ oz butter, soft

- 8 and ½ oz of cream cheese, soft

- 6 tbsp dark cocoa powder

- 2 tsp vanilla + 2 tbsp granulated sweetener

- 2 and ½ oz of walnut pieces

Direction

1. Take a bowl and mix in all ingredients
2. Transfer the mixture to a lined dish
3. Transfer the dish to your fridge and let it chill for 2-3 hours
4. Slice and serve
5. Enjoy!

Per Serving Calories: 124 Fat: 13g Carbohydrates: 2.2g Protein: 2.2g

32 - Candy Caramels

Preparation	Cooking	Servings
4 hours	**6 min**	**8**

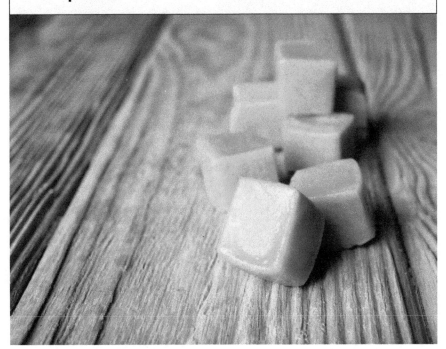

Ingredients

- 2 c of butter

- 4 c of heavy whip cream

- 12 tbsp of stevia powder extract

Direction

1. Take a non-stick saucepan and place it over medium-low heat

2. Add butter and let it melt, heat until light brown

3. Add cream and stevia to butter and paddle for 2 minutes until sticky
4. Remove from heat and keep mixing
5. Pour into candy molds and chill for 3-4 hours
6. Serve and enjoy!

Per Serving Calories: 222 Fat: 41g Carbohydrates: 1.2g Protein: 1.2g

33 - Vanilla Custard

Preparation	Cooking	Servings
15 min	7 min	8

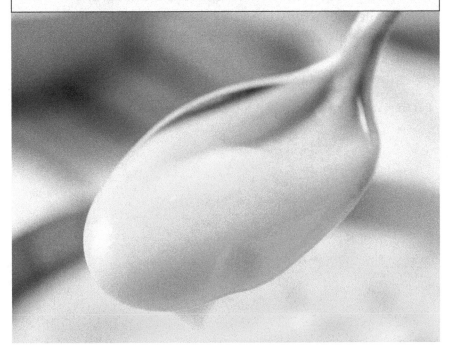

Ingredients

- 12 whole egg yolks
- 1 c of unsweetened almond milk
- 2 tsp of vanilla extract
- 8 tbsp of melted coconut oil
- 2 tsp of stevia

Direction

1. Whisk egg yolks, almond milk, vanilla, and stevia in a medium-sized metal bowl
2. Slowly mix in melted coconut oil and stir
3. Place the bowl over a saucepan of simmer water
4. Keep whisking the mixture vigorously until thick
5. Use a thermometer to register the temperature; once it has reached 140 degrees Fahrenheit, keep it steady for 3 minutes
6. Remove the custard from the water bath and serve chilled!

Per Serving Calories: 214 Fat: 16g Carbohydrates: 7g Protein: 4g

34 - Raspberry and Coco Barks

Preparation	Cooking	Servings
70 min	0 min	8

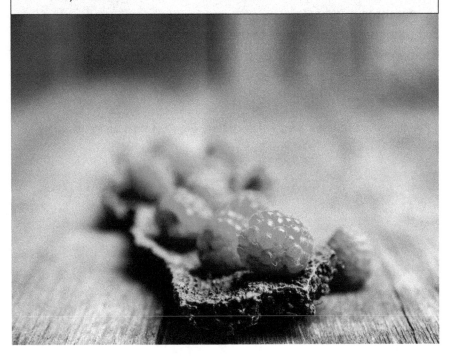

Ingredients

- 1 cup of dried raspberries (frozen)

- 1 cup of coconut butter

- 1 cup of coconut oil

- 1 cup of coconut, shredded

- 1 cup of swerve sweetener, powdered

Direction

1. Power your frozen berries in a food processor
2. Keep the mixture on the side
3. Take a saucepan and place it over medium heat; add remaining ingredients and stir gently until melted
4. Pour half of the pan mixture into the baking pan (lined with parchment paper)
5. Mix in powdered berries to the remaining pan mixture and stir
6. Spoon raspberry mixture over coconut mix in your baking pan
7. Let it chill for 1 hour
8. Serve and enjoy!

Per Serving Calories: 223 Fat: 21g Carbohydrates: 6.2g Protein: 3g

VEGAN AND VEGETARIAN

35 - Tender Coconut and Cauliflower Rice

Preparation	Cooking	Servings
30 min	25 min	8

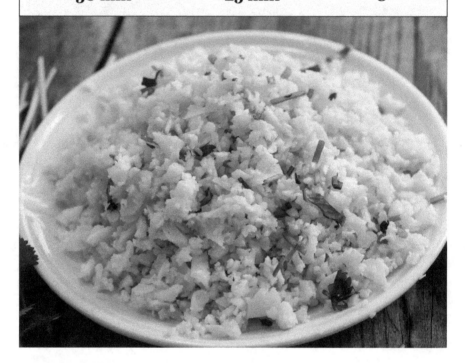

Ingredients

- 6 cups cauliflower, riced
- 3 cups full-fat coconut milk
- 2 teaspoons sriracha paste
- ½ teaspoon onion powder
- Salt as needed
- Fresh basil for garnish

Direction

1. Take a pan and place it over medium low heat

2. Add all of the ingredients and stir them until fully combined

3. Cook for about 5-10 minutes, making sure that the lid is on

4. Remove the lid and keep cooking until any excess liquid goes away

5. Once the rice is soft and creamy, enjoy!

Per Serving Calories: 85 Fat: 6g Carbohydrates: 3g Protein: 1.2g

36 - Almond and Blistered Beans

Preparation	Cooking	Servings
15 min	25 min	8

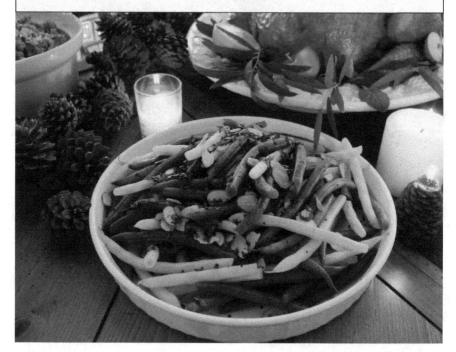

Ingredients

- 2 pound fresh green beans, ends trimmed
- 3 tablespoon olive oil
- 1 teaspoon salt
- 3 tablespoons fresh dill, minced
- Juice of 2 lemon
- 1 cup crushed almonds
- Salt as needed

Direction

1. Pre-heat your oven to 400-degree F

2. Add in the green beans with your olive oil and also with salt

3. Then spread them in one single layer on a large sized sheet pan

4. Roast it up for 10 minutes and stir it nicely, then roast for another 8-10 minutes

5. Remove it from the oven and keep stirring in the lemon juice alongside the dill

6. Top it up with crushed almonds and some flak sea salt and serve

Per Serving Calories: 327 Fat: 18g Carbohydrates: 5g Protein: 25g

37 - Buttery Green Cabbage

Preparation	Cooking	Servings
15 min	20 min	8

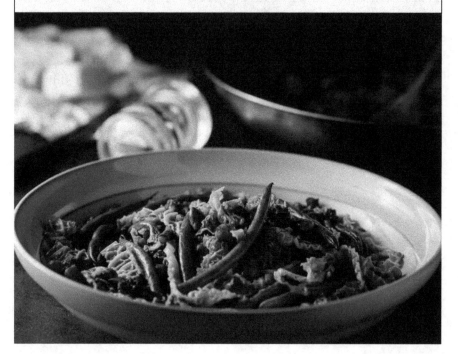

Ingredients

- 3 pounds shredded green cabbage
- 6 ounces butter
- Salt and pepper to taste
- 2 dollop, whipped cream

Direction

1. Take a large skillet and place it over medium heat

2. Add butter and melt

3. Stir in cabbage and Saute for 15 minutes

4. Season accordingly

5. Serve with a dollop of cream

6. Enjoy!

Per Serving Calories: 189 Fat: 16g Carbohydrates: 11g Protein: 3.2g

38 - Lemon and Broccoli Dish

Preparation	Cooking	Servings
20 min	15 min	8

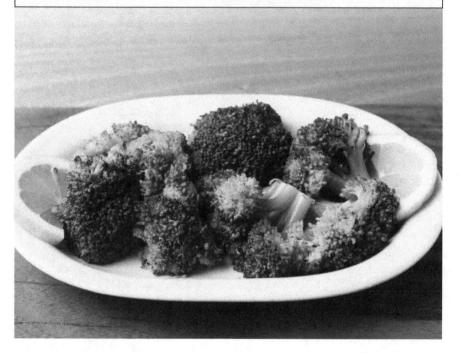

Ingredients

- 4 heads broccoli, separated into florets
- 4 teaspoons extra virgin olive oil
- 2 teaspoon salt
- 1 teaspoon black pepper
- 2 garlic clove, minced
- 1 teaspoon lemon juice

Direction

1. Pre-heat your oven to 400 degree F

2. Take a large sized bowl and add broccoli florets
3. Drizzle olive oil and season with pepper, salt and garlic
4. Spread broccoli out in single even layer on a baking sheet
5. Bake for 15-20 minutes until fork tender
6. Squeeze lemon juice on top
7. Serve and enjoy!

Per Serving Calories: 59 Fat: 2.9g Carbohydrates: 5g Protein: 3.2g

39 - Grilled Veggie Salad with Feta

Preparation	Cooking	Servings
15 min	15 min	8

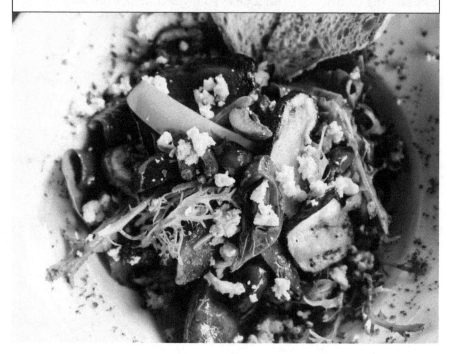

Ingredients

- 6 grilling vegetables of your choice (e.g., eggplant, zucchini, and onions)
- 1 tsp oregano
- 1 cup of crumbled feta
- 4 tbsp of olive oil
- 2 tbsp of balsamic vinegar

Direction

1. In a grilling pan or in the broiler, cut the veggies into slices, season with oregano and salt/pepper, and cook until done for around 15 minutes.

2. Combine the olive oil and balsamic vinegar in a small cup or bowl to make a vinaigrette.

3. Drizzle the vinaigrette over the veggies and top with the crumbled feta pieces and serve

Per Serving Calories: 181 Fat: 12g Carbohydrates: 8g Protein: 8g

40 - Risotto Mushroom

Preparation	Cooking	Servings
15 min	20 min	8

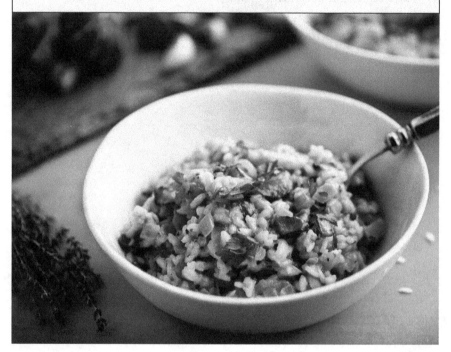

Ingredients

- 2 cup vegetable stock
- 2 head of cauliflower, grated
- 16 ounces mushroom, chopped
- 4 tablespoons butter
- 2 cup coconut cream

Direction

1. Take a saucepan and pour the stock into it

2. Bring it to boil and set it aside
3. Then take a skillet and melt butter over medium heat
4. Add mushroom to sauté until it turns into golden brown
5. Stir in a stock and grated cauliflower
6. Bring the mixture to a simmer and add cream
7. Cook until liquid is reduced and cauliflower is aldente
8. Serve warm and enjoy!

Per Serving Calories: 186 Fat: 16.5g Carbohydrates: 6.7g Protein: 2.8g

REFRESHING DRINKS AND SMOOTHIES

41 - Reishi Pear Smoothie

Preparation	Cooking	Servings
10 min	0 min	4

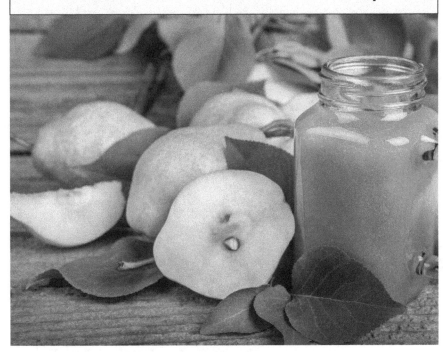

Ingredients

- 1 cup ice
- 2 cup collard greens, chopped
- 2 pear, roughly chopped
- 1 cup raw cashews
- 2 teaspoon reishi mushroom powder
- 2 cup unsweetened cashew milk

Directions

1. Add all the ingredients except vegetables/fruits first

2. Blend until smooth
3. Add the vegetable/fruits
4. Blend until smooth
5. Add a few ice cubes and serve the smoothie
6. Enjoy!

Per serving Calories: 198 Fat: 17g Carbohydrates: 16g Protein: 7g

42 – Lettuce Carrots Smoothie

Preparation	Cooking	Servings
15 min	0 min	4

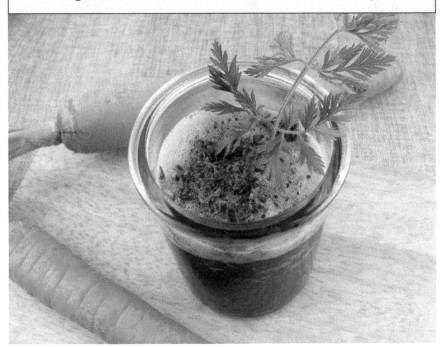

Ingredients

- 1 cup ice
- 10 large leaves romaine lettuce
- 1 cucumber, diced
- 6 celery stalks, chopped
- 2 carrot, shredded
- 2 orange, peeled and segmented
- 1 cup of water

<u>Directions</u>

1. Add all the ingredients except vegetables/fruits first
2. Blend until smooth
3. Add the vegetable/fruits
4. Blend until smooth
5. Add a few ice cubes and serve the smoothie
6. Enjoy!

Per serving Calories: 153 Fat: 1.4g Carbohydrates: 18g Protein: 4.3g

43 - Apple Smoothie

Preparation	Cooking	Servings
10 min	**0 min**	**4**

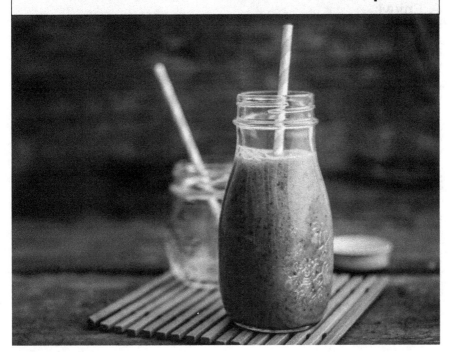

Ingredients

- 1 cup ice
- 3 cups swiss chard, chopped
- 1 cucumber, diced
- 1 grapefruit, peeled and segmented
- 3 small apple, cored and chopped
- 2 scoop collagen protein powder
- 10 mint leaves, chopped
- 2 cup of water

Directions

1. Add all the ingredients except vegetables/fruits first
2. Blend until smooth
3. Add the vegetable/fruits
4. Blend until smooth
5. Add a few ice cubes and serve the smoothie
6. Enjoy!

Per serving Calories: 132 Fat: 1.8g Carbohydrates: 15g Protein: 9g

44 - Sweet Basil Smoothie

Preparation	Cooking	Servings
10 min	0 min	4

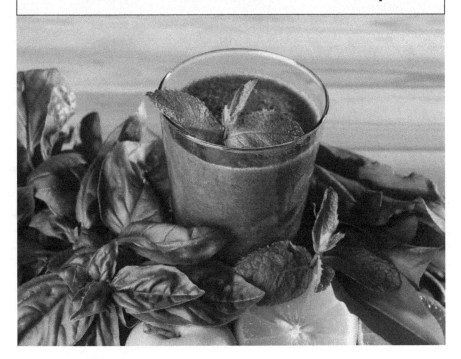

Ingredients

- 1 cup ice
- 2 cup baby spinach, chopped
- 1 cucumber, diced
- 1 cup honeydew melon cubes
- 2 handful basil leaves
- 3 teaspoons ginger, peeled and grated
- Juice of 1 lime
- 2 cup of water

Directions

1. Add all the ingredients except vegetables/fruits first
2. Blend until smooth
3. Add the vegetable/fruits
4. Blend until smooth
5. Add a few ice cubes and serve the smoothie
6. Enjoy!

Per serving Calories: 110 Fat: 2g Carbohydrates: 18g Protein: 3.2g

45 - Purifier Smoothie

Preparation	Cooking	Servings
10 min	0 min	4

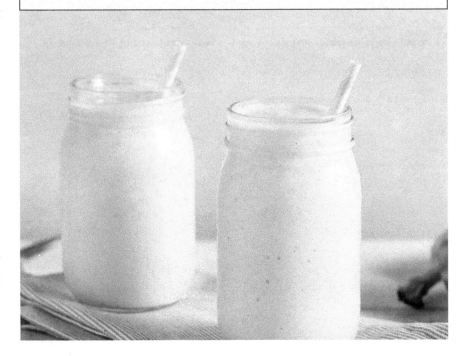

Ingredients

- 1 cup ice
- 10 large leaves romaine lettuce
- 1 cucumber, diced
- 1 cup red bell pepper, chopped
- 2 small Granny Smith apple, cored and chopped
- 2 scoop collagen protein powder
- 10 mint leaves, chopped
- 4 tablespoons fresh-squeezed lemon juice
- 2 cup of water

Directions

1. Add all the ingredients except vegetables/fruits first
2. Blend until smooth
3. Add the vegetable/fruits
4. Blend until smooth
5. Add a few ice cubes and serve the smoothie
6. Enjoy!

Per serving Calories: 170 Fat: 1.4g Carbohydrates: 13g Protein: 20g

46 - Kiwi Cucumber Smoothie

Preparation	Cooking	Servings
10 min	0 min	4

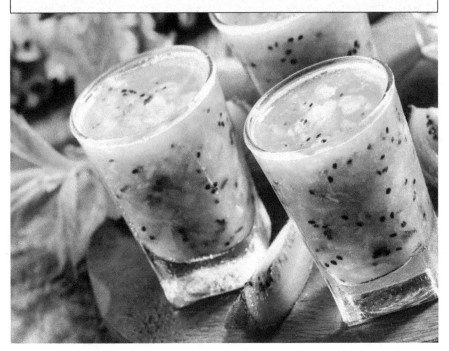

Ingredients

- 2 cup unsweetened cashew milk
- 2 tablespoon lime juice
- 2 tablespoon chia seeds
- 1 cup cucumber, diced
- 1 small green apple, cored
- 2 kiwi, peeled
- 2 cup baby kale, chopped
- 2 cup baby spinach, chopped
- 1 cup ice

Directions

1. Add all the ingredients except vegetables/fruits first
2. Blend until smooth
3. Add the vegetable/fruits
4. Blend until smooth
5. Add a few ice cubes and serve the smoothie
6. Enjoy!

Per serving Calories: 354 Fat: 7.2g Carbohydrates: 12g Protein: 6g

KETO KITCHEN STAPLES AND DISH RECIPES

47 - Buttermilk Dressing

Preparation	Cooking	Servings
15 min	**0 min**	**4**

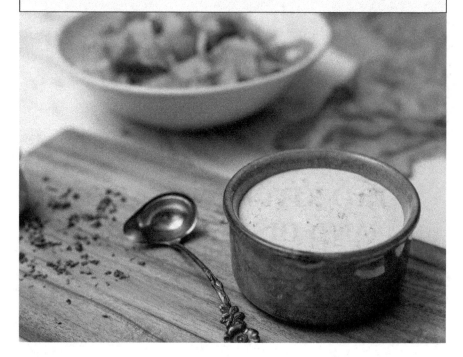

Ingredients

- 4 tablespoons buttermilk
- 1 cup Greek yogurt
- 2 teaspoon apple cider vinegar
- 2 garlic clove, minced
- 2 tablespoon olive oil
- 2 tablespoon fresh parsley leaves

Direction

1. Take a food processor and add butter, milk, yogurt, vinegar, apple cider, garlic, olive oil, parsley and blend well until combined
2. Pour into sealed glass container and chill for 30 minutes
3. Use as needed!

Per Serving Calories: 259 Fat: 24g Carbohydrates: 3g Protein: 3.2g

48 - Spinach Dip

Preparation	Cooking	Servings
15 min	0 min	4

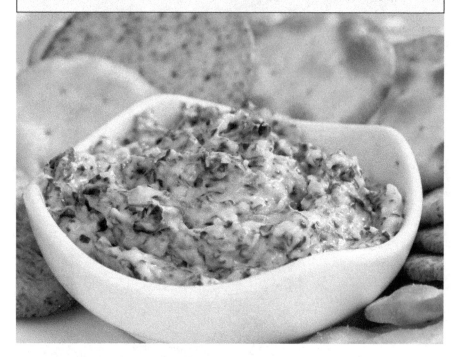

Ingredients

- 20 ounce Spinach, raw
- 3 Greek yogrut
- 2 tablespoon of onion powder
- 1 a teaspoon of garlic salt
- Black pepper to taste
- 1 a teaspoon of Greek Seasoning

<u>Direction</u>

1. Add listed ingredients to a blender and blend well until smooth

2. Season and serve with your desired dipper

3. Enjoy!

Per Serving Calories: 111 Fat: 3g Carbohydrates: 3g Protein: 10g

49 - Béchamel Sauce

Preparation	Cooking	Servings
15 min	10 min	8

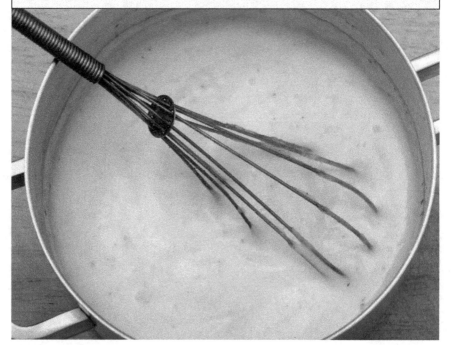

<u>Ingredients</u>

- 3 heavy whip cream
- 4 ounces cream cheese
- 1 teaspoon salt
- 1 teaspoon ground black pepper
- 1 teaspoon nutmeg

Direction

1. Add listed ingredients to a non-stick saucepan and bring to a boil, making sure to keep stirring it continuously
2. Lower heat to low and let it simmer for a few minutes until it reaches your desired consistency
3. Once done, season with salt and pepper and use as needed!

Per Serving Calories: 321 Fat: 81g Carbohydrates: 4.2g Protein: 4.1g

50 - Avocado Mayo Cream

Preparation	Cooking	Servings
15 min	0 min	8

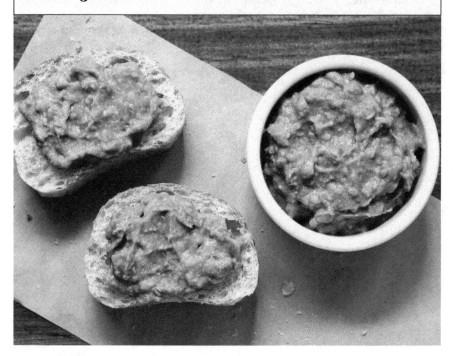

Ingredients

- 2 medium avocado, cut into chunks
- 1 teaspoon ground cayenne pepper
- 4 tablespoons fresh cilantro
- Pinch of salt
- 1 cup olive oil

Direction

1. Take a food processor and add avocado, cayenne pepper, lime juice, salt and cilantro
2. Mix until smooth
3. Slowly incorporate olive oil, add 1 tablespoon at a time and keep processing in between additions
4. Store and use as needed!

Per Serving Calories: 221Fat: 20gCarbohydrates: 4gProtein: 3.2g

CPSIA information can be obtained
at www.ICGtesting.com
Printed in the USA
BVHW092004280521
608095BV00003BA/729